Adult and Paediatric Basic Life Support

Support

CPR and AED

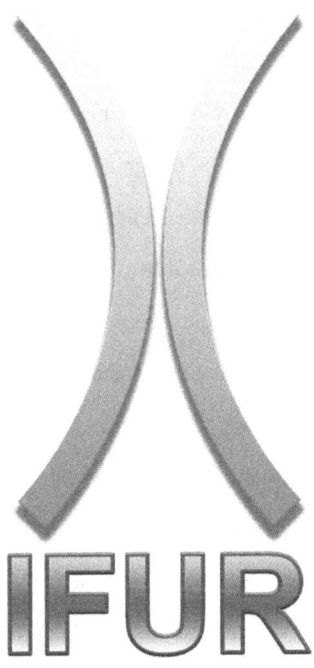

IFUR

Investigación y Formación
en Urgencias

© 2016 José Pérez Vigueras, Ana Laura Barrera Vallejo

© EDITIONS IFUR SL

Edited by Research and Training in Emergency S.L. – IFUR S.L.

C / Obreros Tana 17, 30570, Beniaján – Murcia - España

Ifur@ifur.es

www.ifur.es

ISBN-13: 978-1539786764

ISBN-10: 1539786765

Printed in USA

FIRST EDITION

THANKS

The authors wish to thank our friends and family by I received support in developing this project. And above all,thank Research and Training in Emergency IFUR S.L. confidenceunconditional without which it would have been impossible to develop this project.Thanks to all who have made it possible to develop this guideBasic Cardiopulmonary resuscitation and all management Defibrillatorthe family.

INDEX OF AUTHORS

JOSÉ PÉREZ VIGUERAS Emergency Management. Expert in Emergency and Catastrophes. Instructor Basic and Advanced Life Support - BLS and ACLS by the American Heart Association – AHA

ANA LAURA BARRERA VALLEJO Hospitalization and Emergency nurse. Support Provider Basic and Advanced Vital - BLS and ACLS by the American Heart Association - AHA

PROLOGUE

CARDIAC ARREST is a health problem of the first magnitude, so that this document includes the main issues and changes updating the guidelines of the American Heart Association (AHA) for cardiopulmonary resuscitation (CPR) and Emergency Cardiovascular Emergency (ACE) 2015. It has been developed with the aim that those responsible for resuscitation and AHA instructors have a guide quick reference that provides the basis for these recommendations. Adequate basic training in CPR and in defibrillator management improve the chances of survival for what such knowledge should be included in the basic training those groups as police, health, fire and start school creating potential first responders.

José Pérez Vigueras

INDEX

INTRODUCTION

When we read the figures associated with the rate of death from cardiac arrest we wonder what are higher than these figures, given that in most cases, hands, but are not experts can save lives, and that warning was launched by the Journal of the American Medical Association (JAMA).

However , the figures continue to rise, the day **on October 16** called also the **European Day Cardiac Arrest Awareness** a call of attention on this issue took place, it chilling to think that at least 80% of deaths from cardiac arrest occur in the according ELSEVIER home address.

If we add that information to the above mentioned framework in which those affected are given the most by this disease are far from a hospital environment which leads to a complete misinformation about how to act in such circumstances.

It is for this reason that we deal with this book compiling techniques and alternative means that they can in emergia situation and lack of health professionals trained for realization of cardiopulmonary resuscitation (CPR). So that way we can placate so contudente those situations without giving rise to possible mistakes, here also find the steps you should not do when dealing with potential CPR. So patients as proper development of the possible activity performed.

Is not the whole population should know how to react to a stop?

There is no excuse to not learn CPR and know - how as it is a measure simple, inexpensive and gives results because the important thing is to act at the same time when the stop is given.

For each passing minute chances of survival are reduced in these cases 10%, thereby we realize that immediacy is vital. Each year some 350,000 Europeans suffer from a stop heart outside a hospital setting, but barely 1 in 10 survives.

To conclude this brief introduction, an estimate of the European Resuscitation Council Heart, learn CPR could help save each year around 100,000 life only on the continent.

José Pérez Alcaraz

Health Emergency Technician and Author of the book: First aid for first responders

1. ADULT BASIC LIFE SUPPORT AND CPR QUALITY

The algorithm of BLS in adults has been modified to reflect the fact that rescuers can activate the response system emergencies without departing from the victim (by using a phone mobile).

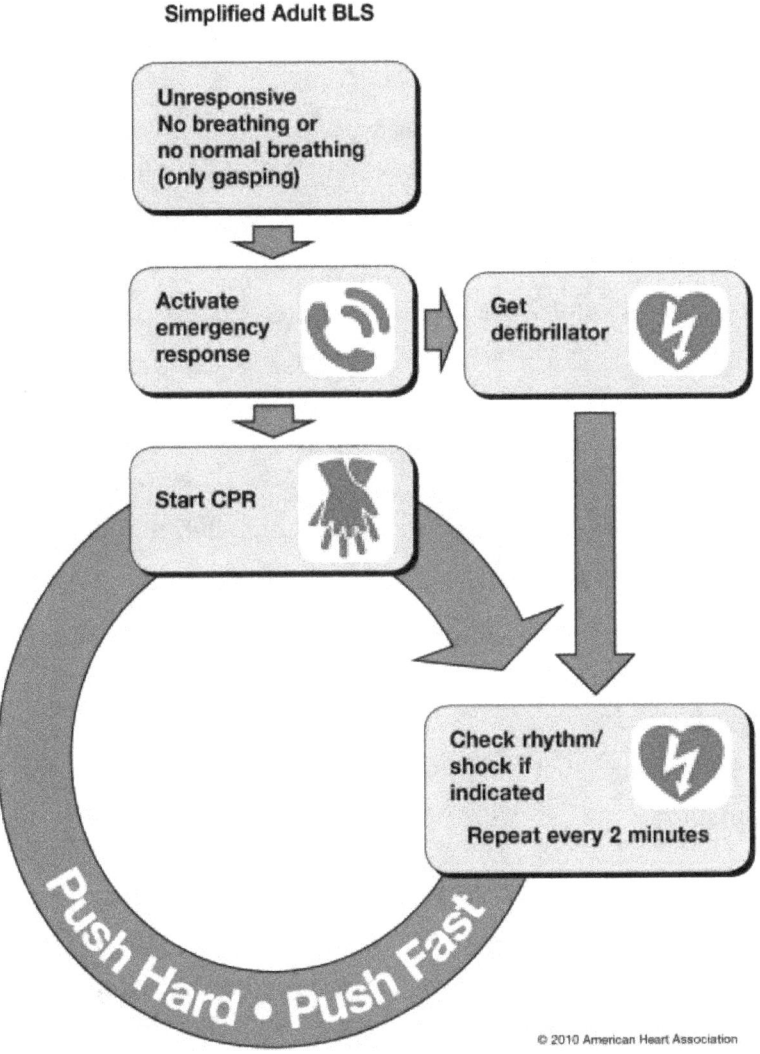

Simplified Adult BLS

© 2010 American Heart Association

PATIENT NOT RESPOND

CPR consists of four main elements:

1. Airway
2. Breathing
3. Circulation
4. Defibrillation

It is important to the immediate recognition of a patient not responds, activating the emergency response system and the start CPR if the lay rescuer notes that the victim does not respond, or it does not breathe normally (eg, pants and gasps).

For one rescuer:

The rescuer has to start chest compressions before practicing the rescue breaths (CAB rather than ABC) to shorten the time until the first compression.

IMPORTANT: You must begin CPR with chest compressions 30/2 ventilations.

1. Stand next to the victim
2. Make sure the victim is lying face up on a firm , flat surface. If the victim is face down, turn with care until your back
3. Aside or remove all clothing covering the chest naked victim needs to be able to see the skin
4. Maneuver front-chin lift:

a. Place one hand on the forehead of the victim and push with the palm to tilt the head back

b. Place the fingers of the other hand under the bony part of the mandibular near the chin

c. Lift the jaw to bring the chin up

d. Quickly open the airway of the victim with the head tilt-chin lift

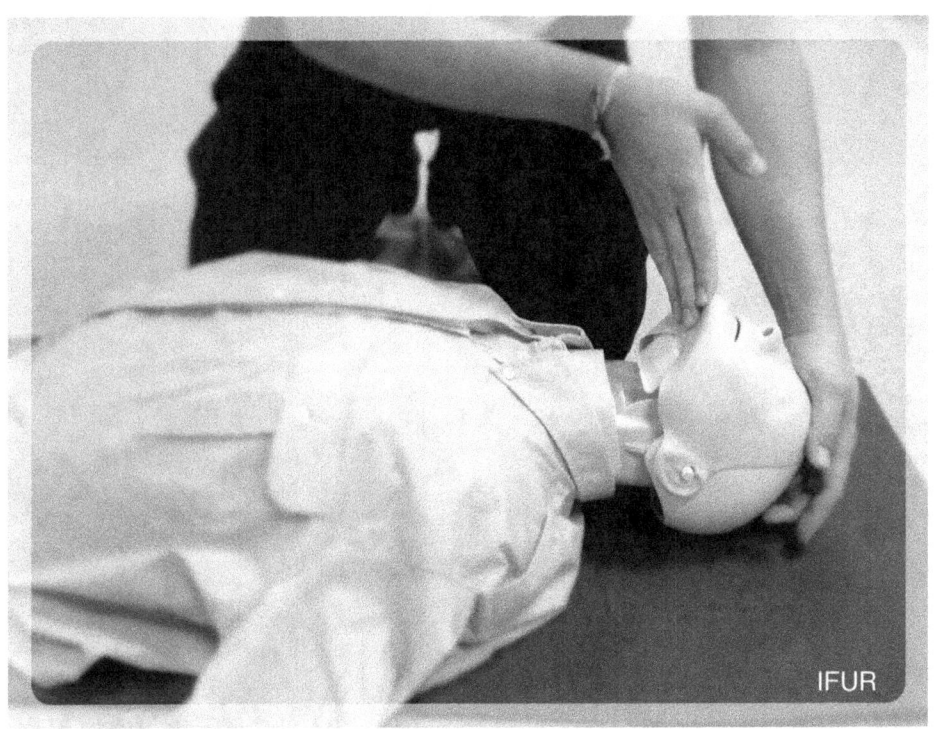

EVALUATION OF THE VICTIM

1. We check the state of consciousness, getting closer to hear the breathing facing the breast

2. Make sure the place is safe for both you and the victim. The idea is that you do not become a victim as well

3. Place the victim on the shoulder and ask loudly: "Are right? "

4. Open the airway of the victim by tilting maneuver head tilt-chin lift

5. Place the ear near the nose and mouth of the victim

6. While looking at the chest of the victim:

    A. See if the chest rises and returns to its position original

    B. Listen for the sound of air breathed

    C. Feel for air comes out against her cheek

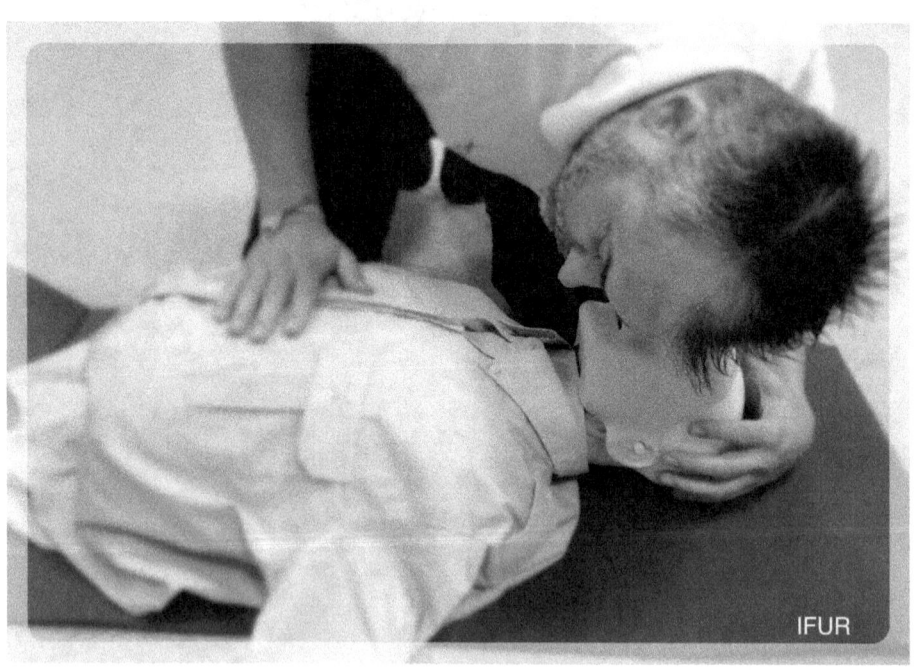

IFUR

We check if the airway is permeable. Ventilate properly, we will perform 2 ventilations after 30 compressions. Each fan will run for 1 second and we ensure that produce chest rise

MOUTH-BREATHING DEVICE BARRIER

1. Stand next to the victim
2. Place the mask over the face of the victim, taking the bridge of the nose as a reference point for correct placement
3. Form a seal between the mask and face
    a. Place the thumb and forefinger of the hand with the highest near the face of the victim on the edge of the mask
    b. Place the thumb of the other hand on her bottom edge the mask
    c. Place the remaining fingers near the neck the victim following the contour of the bones of the jaw and lift. Perform the tilt of the head chin lift to open the airway
    d. As raises The jaw, press Firmly around the outer edge of the mask, for create a tight seal between it and face
4. Breathe normally (not deep) and administer a ventilation (blow for one second). While managing ventilation, observe to make sure the chest rises
5. If the chest does not rise, repeat the maneuver tilt head tilt-chin lift
6. Give a second ventilation (blow for one second). Note to verify that the chest rises

TAKING THE PULSE CAROTID

1.   Keep the nod placing a hand on the front and the victim

2.   Find the trachea using 2 or 3 fingers of the other hand

3.   Slide these 2 or 3 fingers in the groove which lies between the trachea and the lateral muscles of the neck where you can feel the carotid pulse

4.   palpate the artery for at least 5 seconds but not more than 10

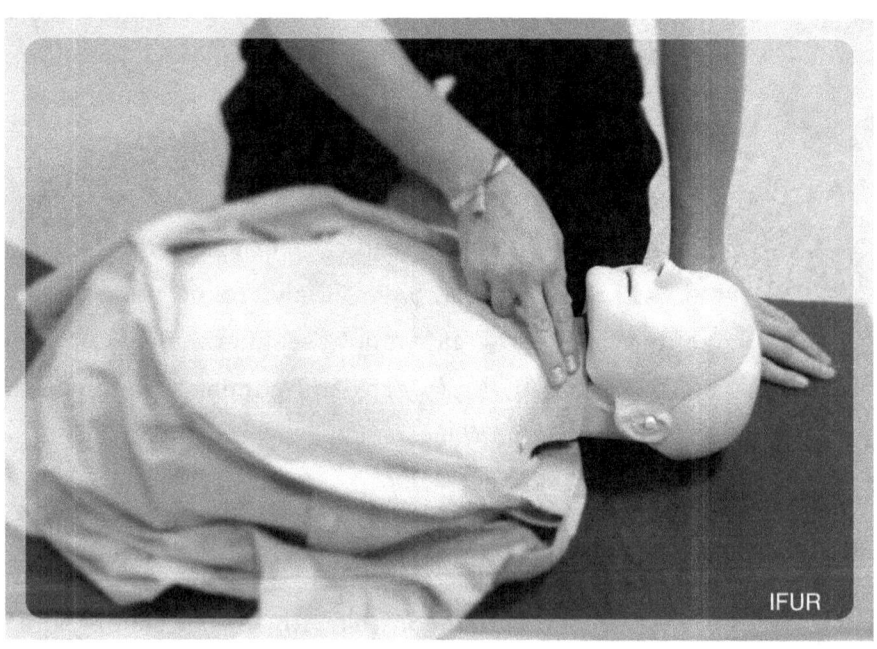

IFUR

CHEST COMPRESSIONS

One of the characteristics of high quality CPR compressions are thoracic and their implementation with adequate rate and depth, allowing complete chest decompression after each compression, minimizing interruptions in compressions and avoiding excessive ventilation.

1. Stand next to the victim
2. Make sure the victim is lying face up on a firm , flat surface. If the victim is face down, turn with care until your back
3. Aside or remove all clothing covering the chest of the victim
4. Place the palm in the center of the bare chest victim between the nipples
5. Place the base of the palm of the other hand over the first
6. Stretch arms and position yourself so that your shoulders are just above their hands
7. Squeeze hard and fast. In each compression sure to be pushing directly on the sternum of the victim
8. After each compression, be sure to allow the chest the victim back to its original position, this will cause the more blood to the heart

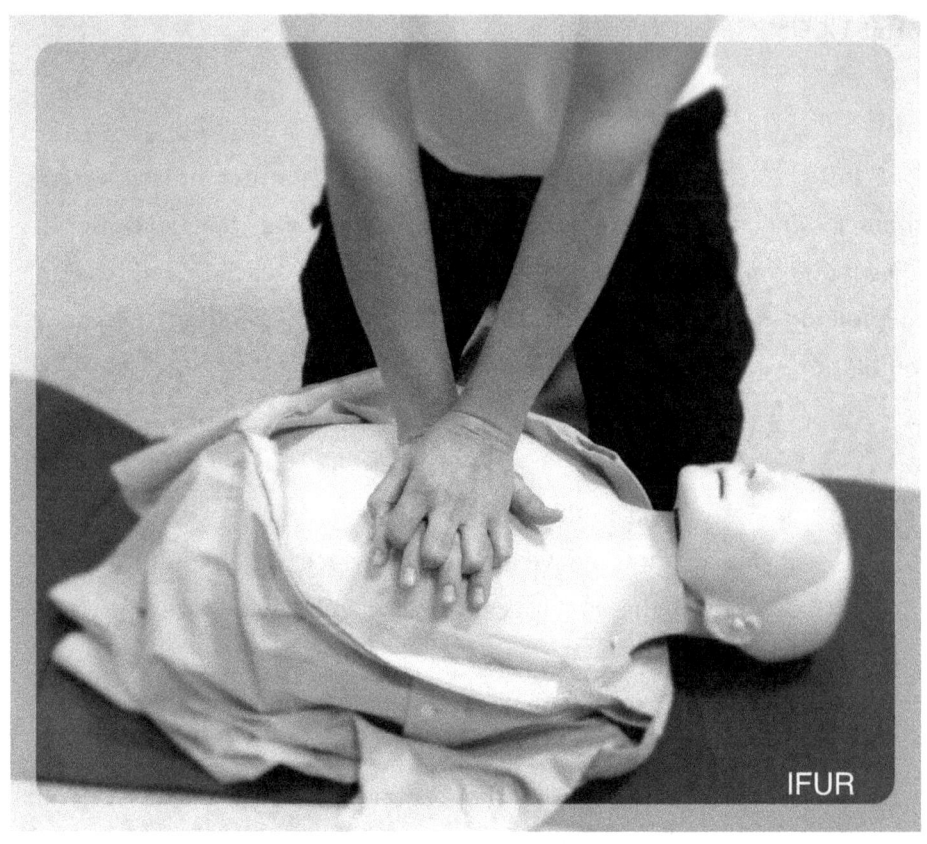

IFUR

The recommended frequency of chest compressions is 100 to 120 cpm.

It is advisable to perform chest compressions rescuers that sink the chest at least one third of the anteroposterior diameter same, at least 5cm. and up to 6cm.

The frequency of compressions for CPR for 2 rescuers is about 120 compressions per minute in adults and 30/2.

Included in those recommendations adolescents, which depending thoracic volume will be performing CPR with one hand or two.

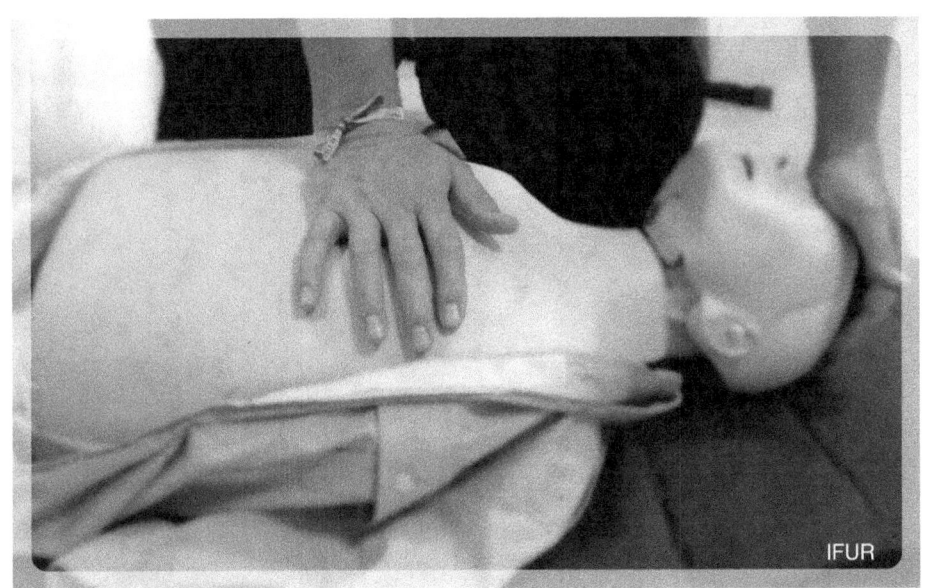

USING THE SYSTEM BAG-MASK

1.   Put on the head of the victim

2.   Put the mask on the face of the victim, taking the bridge of the nose as a reference point for correct placement

3.   Use the technique EC to keep the mask in place while raising the jaw so that the airway remains open

    A. Place the thumb and index finger in a "C" press the edges of the face mask

    B. Place the remaining fingers to lift angles jaw (3 fingers form an "E") and open the airway

4.   Squeeze the bag to give ventilations, each 1 a second, while watching if the chest rises. The administration ventilations is the same with or without supplemental oxygen

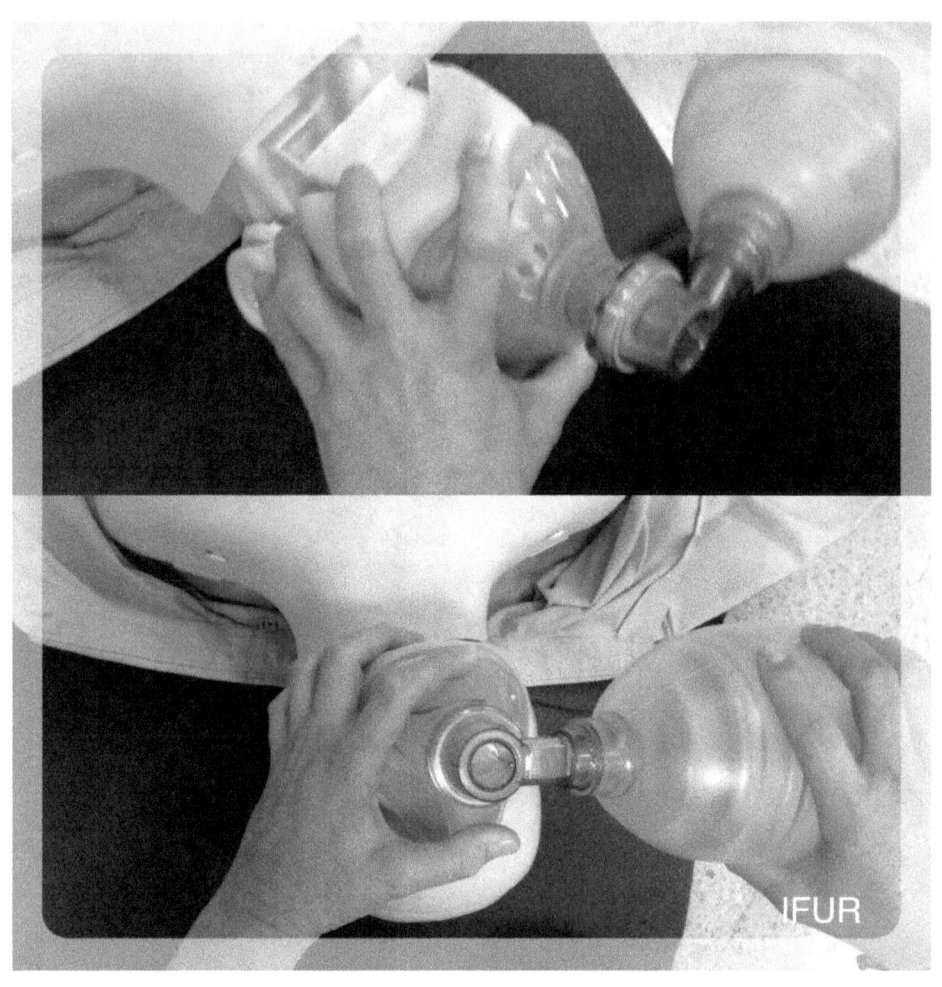

Rescue breathing bag-mask or mask only

Sometimes the victims have inadequate or no breathing They breathe, but if you have a pulse.

In these cases, rescuers administered without ventilations chest compressions. This is called rescue breathing.

RESCUE BREATHING IN ADULTS

1. Administer 1 ventilation every 5 to 6 seconds, about 10 to 12 per minute ventilations
2. Each ventilation should last 1 second
3. Each ventilation should achieve visible chest rise
4. Check the pulse every 2 minutes

Rescuers CPR FOR 2 ADULTS

Rescuer 1. Beside the victim

1. Perform chest compressions
2. Count aloud
3. Turns with the second rescuer every 5 cycles or 2 minutes. He change must be made in less than 5 seconds

Rescuer 2. At the head of the victim

1. Keeps the airway open
2. Manage ventilations, noting that the chest rise and avoiding hyperventilation
3. Encourages the first rescuer to perform compressions what sufficiently frequent and deep and allow the chest return completely to the original position between compressions
4. It turns with the first rescuer every 5 cycles or 2 minutes. He change must be made in less than 5 seconds

INTEGRATION OF CONTENTS

• Assess the victim for unresponsiveness. If you do not respond, shout to ask help

• If you are alone, activate the emergency medical system by Mobile calling 1- 1- 2 and if available get a DESA

• Open the airway of the victim and check breathing, this should occupy at least 5 seconds but not more than 10

• If breathing is inadequate, give two ventilations

• Check the pulse of the victim, this should occupy at least 5 seconds, but not more than 10

• If you are not completely sure he detected pulse, perform five cycles of compressions and ventilations, 30/2 to a rate of 120 / min

2. PEDIATRIC BASIC LIFE SUPPORT AND CPR QUALITY

In pediatric compressions and ventilation SVB sequence are needed C - A - B.

CPR IN INFANTS

The sequence of SVB in infants is:

1.   Airway
2.   Breathing
3.   Circulation

MANEUVER HEAD TILT-CHIN LIFT

1. Place your hand on the forehead of the victim and push the palm to tilt the head back
2. Place the fingers of the other hand under the bony part of the jaw near the chin
3. Lift the jaw to bring the chin forward. The head is in neutral or sniffing

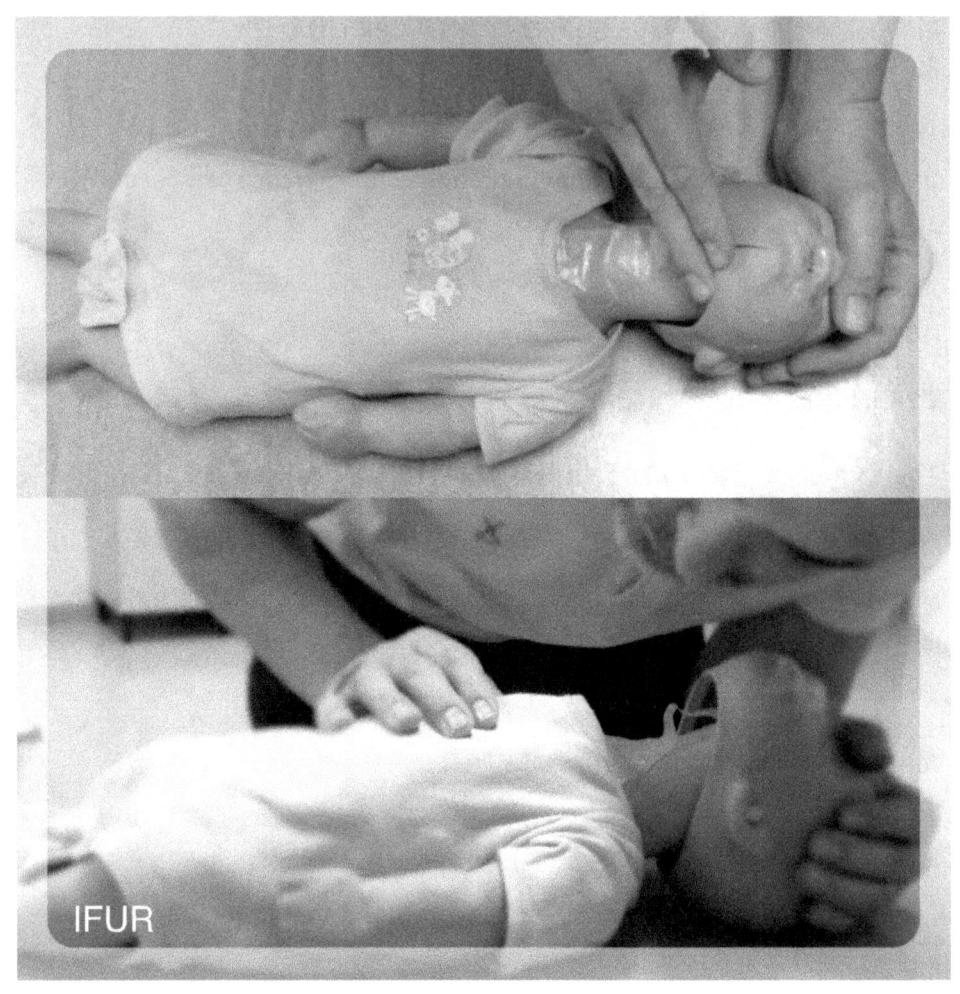

IFUR

MOUTH-BREATHING MOUTH-NOSE AND MOUTH-BREATHING MOUTH

1. Use barrier devices in the same manner as adult victims
2. Keep the head tilt-chin lift for the airway is open
3. Place the mask over the mouth and nose of the infant so as to form an airtight seal

4. Exhale to the nose and mouth of the infant (pausing to breathing between breaths) to make the chest rise with each ventilations

5. If the chest does not rise repeat the above steps until I raised

BREATHING IN INFANTS AND RESCUE

1. Administer 1 ventilation every 3 to 5 seconds (12-20 breaths per minute)
2. Each ventilation should last 1 second
3. Each ventilation should achieve visible chest rise
4. Check the pulse every 2 minutes

TECHNICAL CHEST COMPRESSION

1. Place the infant on a flat surface and firm
2. Remove clothing or covering then remove it from the chest
3. Draw an imaginary line between the nipples. Place 2 fingers on her breastbone just below this imaginary line. this will allow compressions on the lower half of breastbone
4. To do chest compressions, press on the sternum Infant between ⅓ and ½ anteroposterior diameter of the chest
5. After each compression, do not make any pressure on the sternum and allow the chest to return to its original position or expand completely re
6. Manage compressions regularly, with a frequency 120

compressions per minute

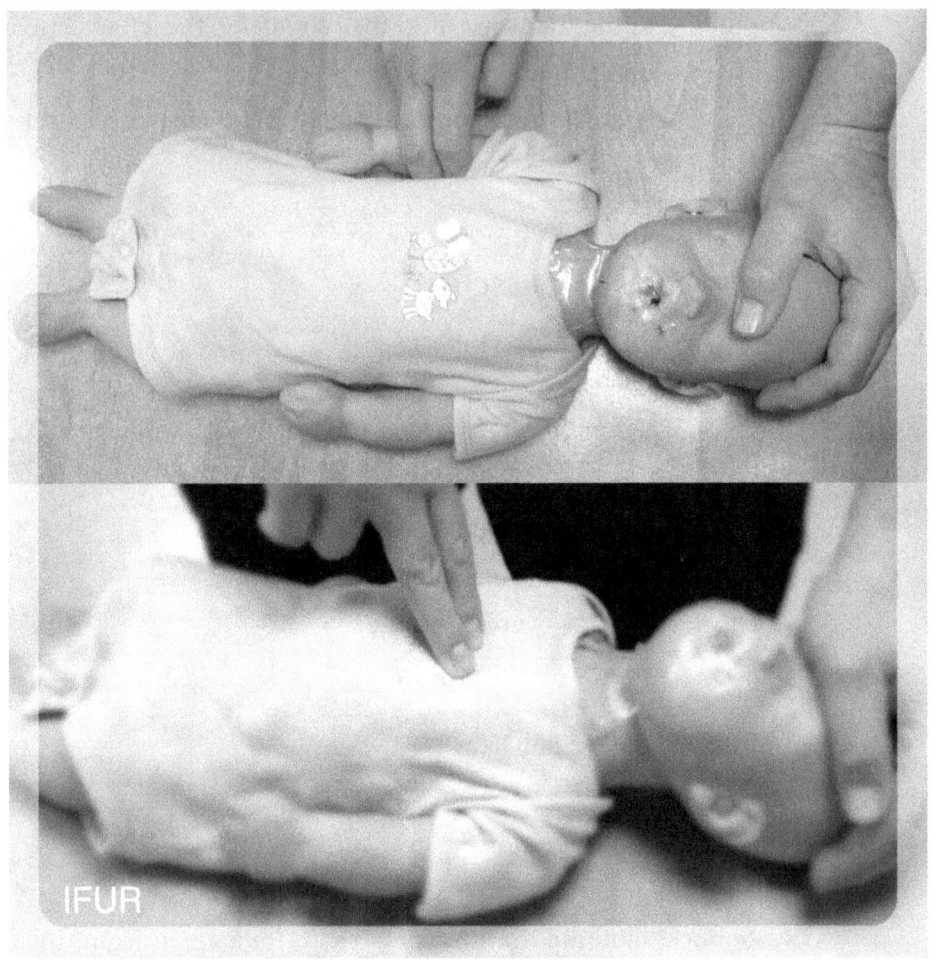

TECHNIQUE TWO THUMBS WITH HANDS AROUND CHEST

1. Draw an imaginary line between the nipples. Place both thumbs, one beside the other, in the center of the lactating breast, on the breastbone just below the imaginary line. this will allow compressions on the lower half of breastbone. Do not perform compressions on the xiphoid. In If the infant is

very small, you can place thumbs each other

2. Encircle the infant's chest and provide back support with fingers of both hands

3. With your hands around the chest, use both thumbs allow the sternum approximately ⅓ and ½ of the diameter anteroposterior chest. While presses down Thumbs, infant chest tighten with fingers

4. After each compression, do not make any pressure on the sternum and allow the chest fully return to its original position

5. Manage compression regularly with a frequency of 120 compressions per minute

6. After 15 compressions, pause briefly for the second rescuer open the airway by tilting the head chin lift and give 2 breaths (the chest should rise with each breath). Coordinate compressions and ventilations to prevent and manage simultaneously order to ensure proper ventilation and chest expansion, especially if the airway is not protected

7. Continue compressions and ventilations with a ratio of 15/2 (for two rescuers) taking turns to perform compressions every 2 minutes CPR sequence by a single rescuer

SEQUENCE 1 RESCUERS CPR FOR INFANTS

1. Assess the victim for unresponsiveness. If you do not respond, shout to request help

2. If someone answers, send that person to activate the system medical emergencies

3. Open the airway of the victim

4. Check the victim's breathing (this should be done at least in 5 seconds, but not more than 10)

5. If the victim has no pulse or heart rate is less than 60 beats per minute with signs of poor perfusion, start cycles compressions and breaths 30/2 with a rate of 120 cpm

SEQUENCE 2 RESCUERS CPR FOR INFANTS

When a second rescuer available to help, the second rescuer activate the emergency medical system or 911 and then return to the victim to help perform CPR. Rescuers They take turns to perform chest compressions changing position every 2 minutes.

Rescuer 1. Beside the victim

1. Perform chest compressions with the technique of the two thumbs with hands around the chest

2. Count aloud

3. turns with the second rescuer every 5 cycles or 2 minutes and the change takes less than 5 seconds

Rescuer 2. At the head of the victim

1. It keeps the airway open

2. Manage ventilations which makes the chest rise

3. Encourages the first rescuer to perform compressions enough frequent and deep and allow the chest to return completely to the position between compressions

4. turns with the first rescuer every 5 cycles or 2 minutes and the change takes less than 5 seconds

The frequency and compression ratio and ventilation during CPR for two Rescuers is 15/2 with a rate of 120 cpm.

In pediatric patients (infants [less than 1 year old] children to the onset of puberty) the depth of compressions should be 1/3 of his ribcage. This equates to approximately 4 cm in infants and 5 cm in children. Once children reach puberty (sI mean, are now teenagers), the depth of compressions is used recommended adult dose of at least 5 cm and at most 6 cm.

EVALUATION OF INFANTS

1. We check the state of consciousness, getting closer to hear the breathing facing the breast

2. Make sure the place is safe for you and for victim. The idea is that you do not become a victim as well

3. Tap the victim in the foot and ask loudly, are you okay?

4. If no response yell for help. If someone comes, send that person to activate the emergency medical system or 911. Then start CPR sequence

5. Open the airway of the victim by tilting maneuver head tilt-chin lift. Be sure to extend the just head back up to the neutral position or sniffing

6. Place the ear near the nose and mouth of the victim

7. While looking at the chest of the victim

8. Observe if the chest rises and returns to its original position

9. Listen for the sound of air breathed

10. Feel if the air strikes against her cheek

11. Manage two ventilations. With a barrier device, give two ventilations with an interval of 1 second to the chest rise

12. Check the brachial pulse.

13. Place 2 fingers on the inside of the arm between the elbow and the infant shoulder

14. Press the inner side arm gently, with the index finger and a half. For at least 5 seconds but not more than 10 seconds.

15. Start cycles of 30 chest compressions and 2 ventilations with a single rescuer and 15/2 with two rescuers, if the infant is still not breathing or pulse is less than 60 lpm

16. The compression depth will be between ½ and ⅓ the diameter chest anteroposterior

17. If you are alone, perform 5 cycles and then activate 30/2 Emergency medical system or by calling 911

In infants and children, begin CPR with chest compressions rather than rescue breaths (C-A-B rather than A-B-C). CPR should begin with 30 compressions (resuscitation by a single rescuer) or with 15 compressions (in resuscitation of infants and children conducted by 2 PS) rather than 2 ventilations.

3. USING THE SEMIAUTOMATIC DESFIBRILATOR – AED

In the case of cardiac arrest in an adult victim with a witness face and immediate availability of an AED, it is reasonable to use the defibrillator as soon as possible. In the case of adult victims They suffer cardiac arrest without monitoring or when no DESA immediately accessible, it is reasonable to start CPR while try to get and apply the defibrillator and defibrillation, if indicated, will try as soon as the device is ready for use.

WHAT IS A AED?

It is a portable device used to stimulate an electrically heart is in ventricular fibrillation. When using an AED are made strong electric shock pass between patches placed on the chest patient. They can be found installed in different places like administrative buildings, gyms, airports, subway stations or rail and will be properly marked.

Most have three simple buttons or steps.

1. Power
2. Analysis heart rhythm
3. Download or electric shock

TYPES OF AED

Defibrillators are computerized, reliable and secure devices that reléase an electric victims of sudden cardiac arrest shock.

They use visual and verbal prompts to guide the actions of the resuscitators and are suitable for use by outsiders world health or health professionals.

Some have a screen where you can visualize the rhythm heart and visual messages.

There are two types of equipment. Most are semiautomatic, this is that to release the electric shock and after recommending it should be the rescuer who with the press of a button performs the download. Others they are fully automatic in which the discharge occurs without specifying resuscitator intervention.

ACTION SEQUENCE IN THE USE OF AED

1. Make sure that both you and the victim and all that around they are safe.
2. If the victim is unresponsive and breathing normally, send someone to for AED and call 911
3. Start maneuvers basic CPR and heart massage Word of mouth ventilations, with a sequence of 30/2 with a rhythm120 cpm
4. As soon as the defibrillator arrives: turn it on and place adhesive electrodes

5. If more than one rescuer should continue CPR while it prepares

6. Follow the verbal or visual instructions

7. Make sure that nobody touches the victim while the AED analyzes the rhythm

8. Act as directed by AED. If a shock is indicated

9. Make sure that nobody touches the victim

10. Press the shock following the signs

11. Follow the visual or verbal instructions

12. If a shock is not indicated, resume immediately PCR, using a ratio 30:2

13. Follow the visual or verbal instructions

14. Follow the instructions in the AED until:

    A. Arrive professional help and relieve resuscitation

    B. The victim starts breathing normally

    C. is exhausted

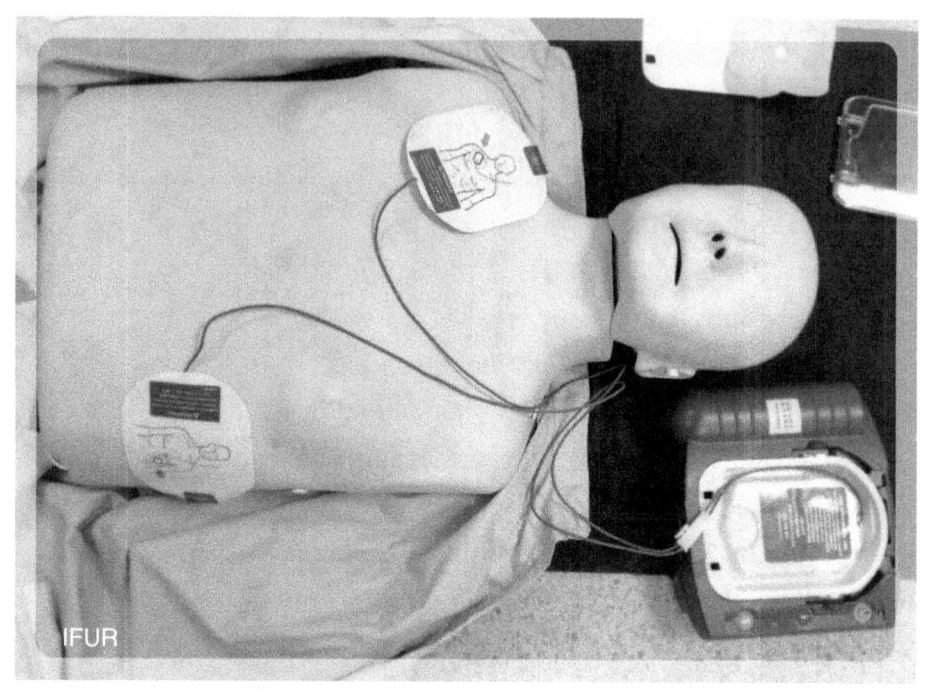

PLACEMENT OF DESA PATCHES

The chest of the victim must be fully exposed to achieve Proper placement of the patches. Chest hair may prevent adhesion patches and interfering electrical transmission. Should a patch placed on the chest to the right of the breastbone

below the collarbone. The other should be placed at the level of the axillary line

half left upright of its longest axis. Women should Avoid placement over the breasts.

Although the vast majority of patches are marked right and left, or have a figure indicating the correct position, is not altered operation if placed in reverse.

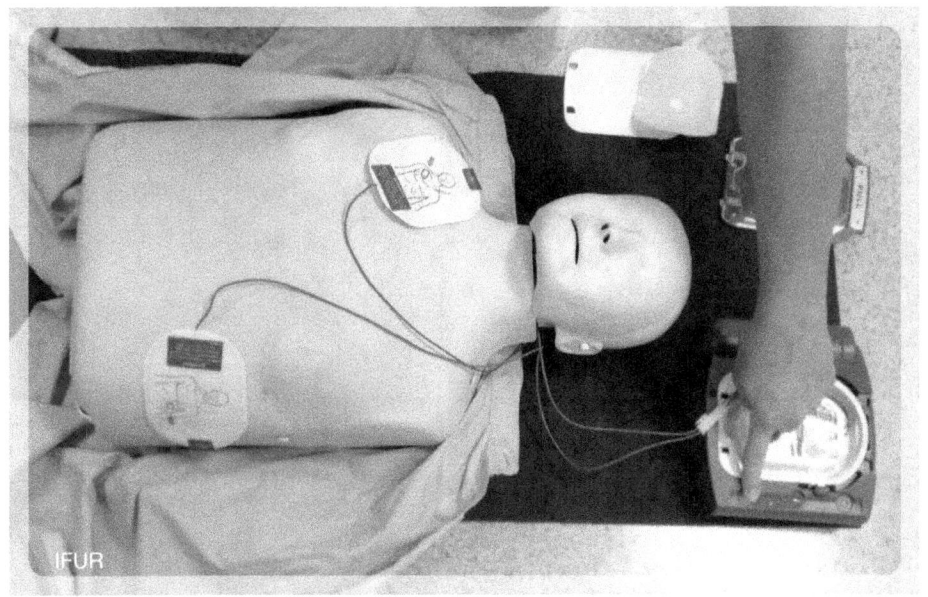

SPECIAL SITUATIONS IN THE USE OF AED

The following five special situations may require persons AED use any additional work .

The victim is younger than 1 year old

At present there is insufficient evidence to recommendation for or against the use of AED in infants children under 1 year of age.

The victim has a lot of chest hair

1. If the patches adhere to hair instead of skin, press them hard
2. If the AED continuous warning that "the patches check", remove patches quickly. This removes a significant amount of hair
3. If still remains a significant amount of hair in place where it should be placed patches, shave the area with razor
4. Place a new patches and follow the verbal instructions of AED

The victim is submerged in water or have wet chest

Water is a good conductor of electricity. Do not use the AED in Water. If the victim is in the water, remove the place. If the chest victim is wet, water can conduct electricity discharge through the chest skin. This prevents the administration of a dose of appropriate shock to the heart. In the event that the victim's chest is wet, dry quickly before connecting the patches. If the victim lying on the snow or small puddle, you can use the AED.

The victim has implanted a pacemaker or defibrillator

You can identify it by being a lump the size of a box and it has a small scar. If it identifies:

1. Place the patch AED at least 2.5 cm away from device

2.   Follow the normal sequence of AED

The victim is a transdermal patch

Do not place AED patches directly over a patch medication. Remove and clean the area before connecting the patch AED SELECT patches AED OR PEDIATRIC SYSTEM Some are designed to deliver AED dose downloads suitable for adults and children. If you are using an AED on a child AED and that can deliver a shock to pediatric doses, follow the AED instructions to select the download with the lowest dose (Pediatric). You may need to press a button or place a switch pediatric mode or use patches for children or both, to reduce the dose of the download. Must be careful not to administer a pediatric download victims over 8 years of age as a lower doses may not be effective in larger victims or age.

If you use an AED on a child aged 1 to 8 years old and lacks AED patch for children or a switch to activate the pediatric mode, you can use the patches for adults and a dose for Adults. 8 years of age and older Use only patches for adults. Do not use patches or button or system switch pediatric victims 8 years of age or greater.

1 to 8 years old

If available, use pediatric pads. If not available, you can use patches adults, provided they do not touch each other , placing one in the front of the chest and the other in the part later. If the AED has a button or switch functions to manage a dose of pediatric download, activate it.

CPR BEFORE DEFIBRILLATION

Immediate defibrillation as soon as it has a AED, is a and it is considered a key element of paramount importance to survive a cardiac arrest due to ventricular fibrillation. However, a period of chest compressions before defibrillation and while it has the defibrillator near the victim, can improve survival.

VOICE MESSAGES

In most devices, the actuation sequence specifies "follow voice instructions/visual". Generally, these can be program, and it is recommended to be determined according to the sequence shocks and CPR times.

INTEGRATION OF CONTENTS

1.   Evaluate the victim for unresponsiveness. If you do not respond, shout to ask help

2.   If someone answers, send email to activate the emergency system   medical and get a AED

3.   Open the airway of the victim and evaluate breathing (this should   occupy him at least 5 seconds, but not more than 10)

4.   If the victim is not breathing give 2 ventilations (may pair need several attempts to open the airway and give 2 vents that make the chest rise)

5.   Check the pulse of the victim, you must employ at least 5 seconds   but not more than 10.

6.   If the victim has no pulse begin CPR. Perform cycles compressions and ventilations, with a frequency ratio of 30/2 120 compressions per minute

7.   After 5 cycles of CPR

8.   If no one has done, activate the emergency medical system and get a   AED

9.   Use the AED

4. SPECIAL CIRCUMSTANCES OF RESUSCITATION

Safety at emergency

When administering CPR, first verify that the site of the emergency It is safe. For example, if a person who needs resuscitation Located near a building that is burning in or near wáter electrical cables, first make sure that both you and the victim are in a safe place.

In case of injury, do not move the victim unless necessary to ensure the safety of the victim or his own.

Rescuer safety

The risk of contracting an infectious disease during CPR is very low. Most hospital cardiac arrest in infants and children occur at home. If the victim suffers from a disease infectious, it is likely that family members have already been exposed to that disease or are aware of it and have barrier devices suitable.

Standard precautions

The administration requires personnel health teams take Standard precautions at work, though they may be exposed to contact with blood or other body fluids. Standard precautions include the use of barrier devices or bag-mask systems, gloves and glasses or goggles

5. SAFETY LATERAL POSITION

1. Stand to the side of the victim
2. Extend the arm closest to you victim above his head, bending the elbow at a right angle
3. Cross the other arm over his chest, placing the back of the hand near the face
4. Bend the leg away from you, leaving your foot resting on soil
5. Turn the victim until his side, leaving the head resting on the arm with the back of the other hand supported on the face
6. Place the victim's head back in a position where keeps the airway open
7. Check the victim's breathing often (Observe, listen and feel)
8. If breathing stops, get a AED, turn the victim until his back and begin CPR

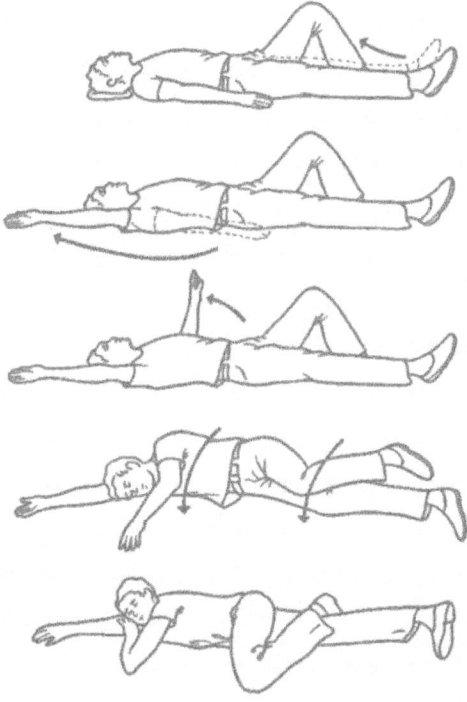

6. CHOKING/OVACE

Choking happens when someone is suddenly blocked by air, where it must pass air and can not breathe. Can be caused due to poor swallowing food or binding objects.

TYPES OF CHOKING

The type of action to reverse must be different if it is a Choking partial or total Choking is therefore the first is to recognize each case:

> • **Choking part:** we realize that the roads are not They are completely blocked because the person will coughing and making noises and hear his labored breathing. It will be hands to her throat, choking unequivocal sign

> • **Total choking:** The person can not make a noise and the foreign object will not allow entry or exit of air. Usually the victim is unable to breathe, your skin starts to pale at first and then becomes colored blue, can shake and lose consciousness. Without attention right may die

The major complication of choking not attend properly is death, but we must also be careful with Partial choking, because they can worsen and pass total, which they are more dangerous.

WHAT TO DO BEFORE A CHOKING

First you have to assess whether it is a partial or total obstruction with above criteria:

In case of partial obstruction: if the person is coughing, you should not interfere, coughing is a defense mechanism to help you expel the foreign object, it is best to encourage him to continue coughing.

In case of total obstruction: The victim no sound, but aware. In this case will be held the Heimlich maneuver, which compressions is try to take the object and smothering unlock the exit and entry of air. The technique to realize it is the following:

1. Stand behind the person while you were standing
2. Put your arms around the waist: his right hand in the form fist closed in the upper abdomen of the person affected (at the level of the stomach, where they join the ribs), and the left hand by taking his fist, surrounding the chest arms base
3. Compress the sudden and strongly belly up with both hands
4. Suspends compression
5. Repeat the maneuver as many times as necessary until the person expels the foreign body from her throat or lose knowledge
6. If you are unconscious, immediately ask for help on the phone 911 emergency, short and clearly communicating happened and begins CPR

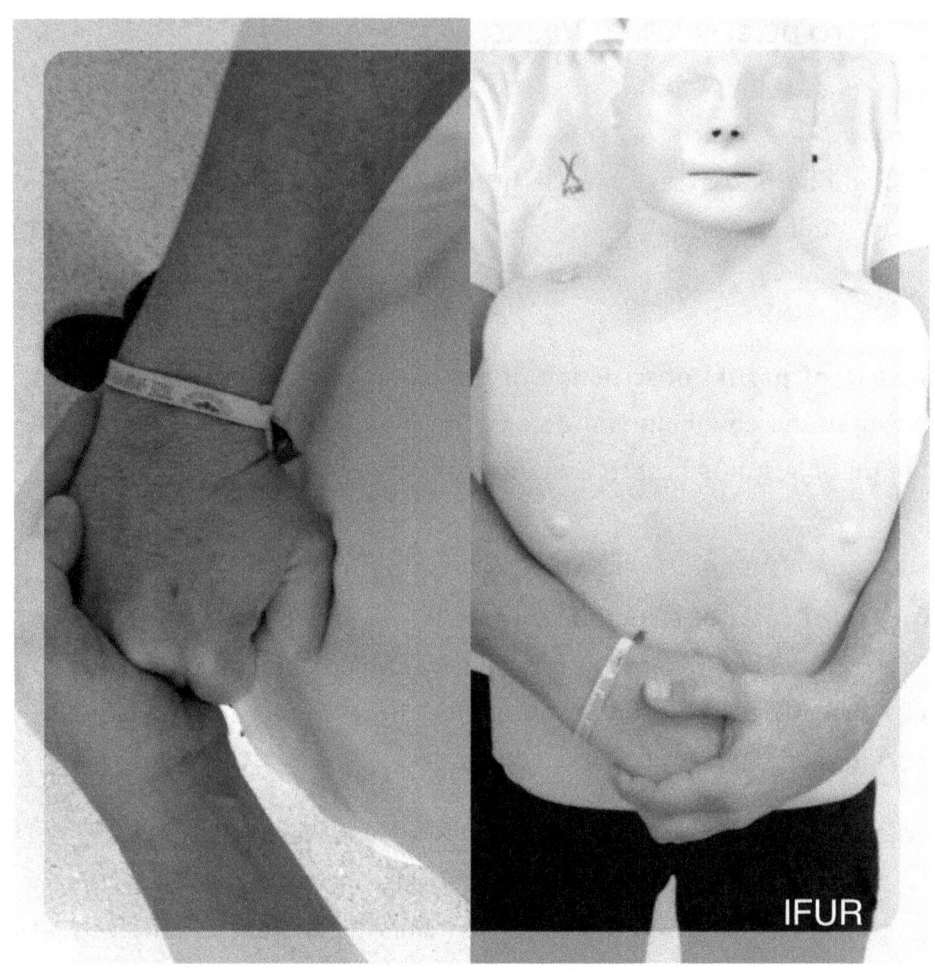

In children older than one year the same procedure is used, but the fist is placed on the child's navel with the thumb side to the abdomen.

RELIEF IN INFANTS WITH ANSWER CHOKING

To remove a foreign body airway of an infant is required a combination of back slaps and punches compressions dry in the chest. To relieve choking in an infant with response, follow the following steps.

1. Kneel or sit and place the infant on her lap
2. If you can do easily, remove the clothes cover the infant's chest
3. Hold the infant with the forearm, prone (face below), with the head at a height slightly lower than the chest. Hold the infant's head and jaw hand. Be careful to avoid compressing the soft tissue of the throat infant. Place the forearm so that it is supported on your lap or thigh, in order to support the infant
4. Manage up to 5 pats on the back vigorously in middle of the back, between the shoulder blades infant, using the base of the palm. Give each claps with enough force to try to remove the foreign body
5. After administration of up to 5 pats on the back, place your hand her free in the back of the infant, I provided support to the back of the infant's head with the palm of his hand. The infant will be adequately accommodated between forearms rescuer, with the palm of one's hands it holding my head and jaw, while the palm of the other hand hold on the back of the head infant
6. Turn the infant so that your body is a unit, care put up with head and neck. Hold the infant face up, with his forearm on his thigh. Keep your head infant to a height less than the trunk
7. Give up to 5 compressions with dry thrusts to the thorax fast and in a downward direction at the same point that perform chest compressions just below the line nipples. Manage compressions with dry thrusts to the thorax at a frequency of one per second, each with intended to provoke an "artificial cough" capable of removing strange body

8. Repeat the sequence up to 5 pats on the back and up to 5 compressions with dry thrusts to the chest until you remove the foreign body or the infant loses consciousness

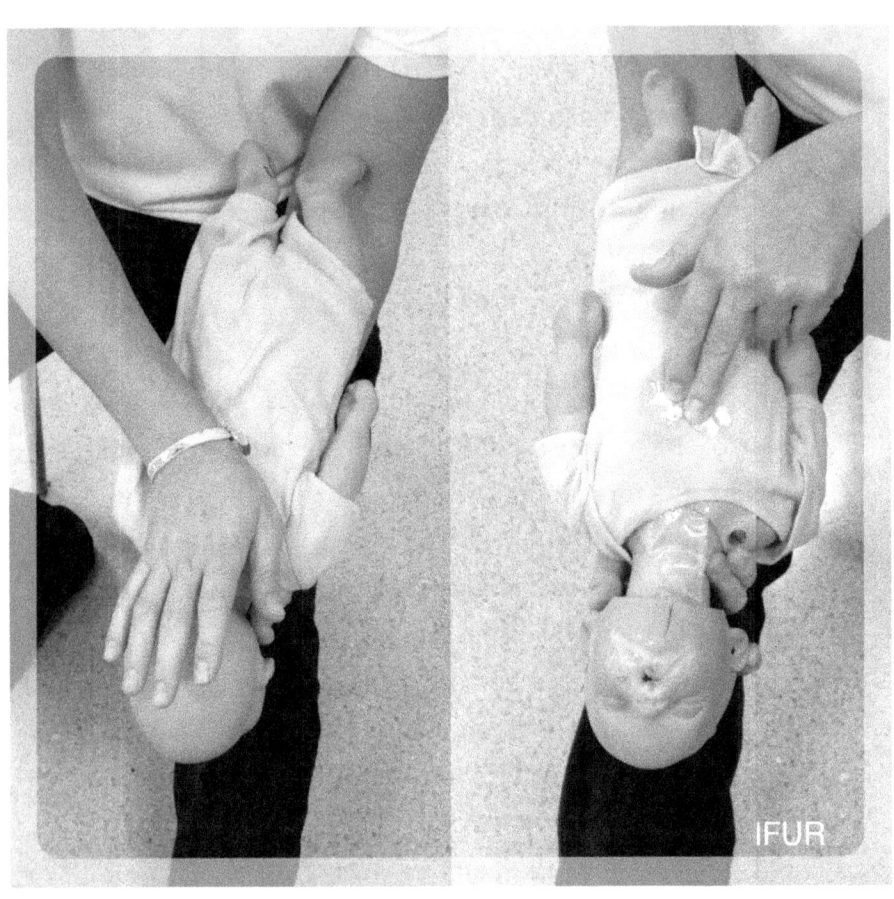

AUTOHEIMLICH

If a person is alone and suffers from drowning by objects that obstruct airway, you can use the Heimlich maneuver on oneself, nailing or placing the weight on the back of a chair, Thus the pressure in the chest is increased rapidly, forcing the object to get out of the airway.

ATAGANTAMIENTO IN OBESE OR PREGNANT WOMEN VICTIMS

If the victim is pregnant or obese, perform compressions with punches dry in the chest rather than quick abdominal thrusts.

7. CEREBRAL ICTU

ICTU is a cerebrovascular disease that affects vessels that supply blood to the brain. he is also known as stroke (CVA), stroke or thrombosis. The two last terms, however, are more concerned with either different causes of ICTU. ICTU occurs when a blood vessel that carries blood to the brain breaks or is clogged by a blood clot or other particle. Because this rupture or blockage, part of the brain does not get the blood flow needs to. The consequence is that nerve cells in the brain área affected receive no oxygen, so they can not function and die after a few minutes.

CAUSES

Many of the factors that can increase the chances of suffering it can not be controlled (age, family medical history, the race or sex). However, most of the factors that increase the risk can be changed, treated or modified.

- Advanced Age: 55 years past, doubles every decade lived risk of ICTU. However, this does not mean that young people do not suffer the problem
- Sex occur more or less the same amount of ICTU in the two sexes. However, more than half of the deaths are in women
- Family and Inheritance race: the risk of ICTU is higher if someone in the family has suffered. Blacks have more risk of death and suffering greater disabilities tan white, partly because

this race blood pressure high is more prevalent, and this problem is a factor ICTU important risk

- Having suffered a ICTU recently: I had one once the chances of suffering another increase significantly
- Having high blood pressure: Hypertension is the risk factor that best predicts stroke. 70 percent of ICTU occur because of hypertension
- Smoking: in recent years studies have shown that smoking Cigarette smoking is a major risk factor. Nicotine and carbon monoxide damage the cardiovascular system. The use of oral contraceptives plus smoking greatly increases As the risk of ICTU
- Having Diabetes Mellitus: it is an independent risk factor and It is largely related to high blood pressure. Although diabetes can be treated, getting it increases the risk ICTU
- Suffer carotid artery disease. The carotid arteries neck provide blood to the heart. A carotid damaged by Atherosclerosis can block the vessel and cause a clot blood, which can cause a ICTU
- Present heart disease: a diseased heart increases risk of ICTU. Indeed, people with problems heart are twice as likely to develop this problem
- Suffer attacks ischemic transient: produce symptom Similar, but no damage that last
- Meter high red blood cell: a moderate increase or important number of red blood cells also is an indicator ICTU important. The reason is that RBCS cause thickens the blood, which can cause clots more easily
- Season and climate: ICTU deaths occur more often with extremely cold temperaturas hot
- Drinking alcohol in excess: can increase the Pressure blood, increasing obesity, triglycerides, cancer and other disease,

cause heart failure ...

- Certain types of drug use: injecting drug taking intravenous increases the risk of ICTU due to a stroke cerebral. Cocaine use has also been linked strongly to ICTU, attacks from heart and various complications cardiovascular

SYMPTOM

In general, ICTU are sudden onset and rapid development, and cause brain injury in minutes (ICTU established). Less frequently, a stroke can worsen over hours, even for one or two days, as will increasing necrosing tissue área brain (ICTU in evolution). Usually, this progression usually interrupted, but not always, leading to periods of stability in the area of necrotic tissue stops growing transiently or that some improvement is observed.

Depending on the affected area of the brain may occur many different symptoms.

- Sudden numbness or weakness of the face, arm or leg, especially on one side of the body
- sudden confusion, trouble speaking or understanding
- Sudden trouble walking, dizziness, loss of balance or coordination
- Sudden trouble seeing in one or both eyes
- Sudden severe headache with no known cause that

When ICTU affects the left brain region, the affected part body will be right (and left of the face) and may give some or all of the following symptoms:

- Paralysis of the right side of the body
- Speech or language
- Cautious style of behavior, slowed down
- Memory loss If, however

the affected part is the right brain region, will be the left side of the body which have problems:

- Paralysis of the left side of the body
- Vision problems
- Inquisitive behavior, accelerated
- Memory loss

They have developed some ways to know when a person will suffering a ICTU. Among them is, for example, the Cincinnati scale, it is consisting of three tests:

- Facial Asymmetry: the patient is smiling to see if both sides of the face move symmetrically. In case abnormal, one side would show deficiencies to move
- Arm strength: the patient indicates that stretch your arms for 10 seconds. In abnormal case, one of the arms is not moves or falls over the other

49

- Language: the patient to talk indicated. In abnormal case, slurred speech, has trouble speaking or speak

If any of these three checks obtains the abnormal result, it the possibility that the patient will suffer a ICTU.

- Quickly recognize the signs and symptoms of ICTU, scoring when they occur for the first time. Quickly activate services emergency
- Rapid emergency transport to hospital and pre-notification
- Lead patients to a ICTU unit, medical centers specializing in the treatment of this disease
- Start care and patient assessment during the transportation to the hospital: as soon as the patient suffers a ICTU, the responsible medical services should take into account certain aspects of the patient as adequate oxygenation and power controls, blood pressure, blood sugar, fever or other complications
- Receive quickly diagnosis and treatment in hospital so that it is under intensive monitoring

Sometimes must resort to surgery to remove the clot blocks the arteries of the brain.

When the ICTUS has passed, treatment depends on the disabilities who have been to the patient.

MAIN ABBREVIATIONS

AED. semi-automatic / automatic defibrillator

Dm. Mellitus diabetes

Fx. Fracture

Phr. Cardiorespiratory arrest

Slp. Safety lateral position

Pr. Respiratory arrest

Rcp. CPR

SVA. Advanced Life Support

BLS. basic life support

Tac. computed tomography

Tce. Traumatic brain injury

Tto. Treatment

Tx. Trauma / Trauma

PS. Health personnel

V.o. Oral

ICTU. Cerebrovascular disease

REFERENCE

1. Pérez Vigueras, J. Barrera Vallejo, AL. Adult and Pediatric Basic Life Support - CPR and management Semi-Automatic defibrillator – AED. Murcia. ED. IFUR 2015

2. Pérez Vigueras, J. Barrera Vallejo, AL. First Aid for teachers and parents. Murcia. Ed. IFUR 2015

3. 2015 AHA Guidelines for CPR and ECC

4. Pérez Alcaraz, J. Pérez Vigueras, J. Barrera Vallejo, AL. First Aid for First Responders. Murcia. Ed. IFUR 2015

5. Pérez Vigueras, J. Abrisqueta Garcia. J. Barrera Vallejo, AL Manual management, mobilization and transportation of victims. Murcia. Ed. IFUR 2015.

6. Pérez Vigueras, J. Barrera Vallejo, AL. My friend extinguisher. Murcia. Ed. IFUR 2015.

7. Neumar RW, Shuster M, Callaway CW, et. al. Part 1: executive summary, 2015 American Heart Association Guidelines Update for Cardiopulmonary Resuscitation and Emergency Cardiovascular Care. Circulation. 2015

8. Neumar RW, Shuster M, Callaway CW, et al. Part 1: executive summary: 2015 American Heart Association Guidelines Update for Cardiopulmonary Resuscitation and Emergency Cardiovascular Care. Circulation. 2015;132(18)(suppl 2). En prensa

9. Hazinski MF, Nolan JP, Aicken R, et al. Part 1: executive summary: 2015 International Consensus on Cardiopulmonary Resuscitation and Emergency Cardiovascular Care Science With Treatment Recommendations. Circulation. 2015;132(16)(suppl 1). En prensa

10. Nolan JP, Hazinski MF, Aicken R, et al. Part 1: executive summary: 2015 International Consensus on Cardiopulmonary Resuscitation and Emergency Cardiovascular Care Science With

Treatment Recommendations. Resuscitation. En prensa

11. Institute of Medicine. Strategies to Improve Cardiac Arrest Survival: A Time to Act. Washington, DC: National Academies Press; 2015.

12. Pérez Vigueras J. Juárez Torralba J. et al. First involved in the emergency and hospital emergency. Advanced Life Support. Madrid. Aran editions, 2010.

13. Abrisqueta Garcia, J. Juarez Torralba J. Pérez Vigueras, J. Basic Manual management, mobilization and transportation of victims, injured and traumatized. Madrid. Aran editions, 2001.

14. Monteagudo Soto E., Pérez Vigueras, J. Evacuation and transfer of patients. Barcelona. Ed. Altamar, 2012.

15. Pérez Vigueras J. and others. Emergency Manual and Emergency Nursing. Murcia. Ed. Official College of Nursing of Murcia.

16. P. García Pradillo Pharmacology in nursing. Madrid. Ed. DAE, 2003.

17. Vigueras Pérez, J. Perea Lifante, Campillo FJ Pérez, JA Pérez Gracia, JM. I want to be a firefighter 2 - agenda of oppositions. Murcia. Ed. IFUR 2015

18. OPERATION WITH A SINGLE DUMP rescuer. Pérez Vigueras, J. Juarez Torralba, J. Abrisqueta Garcia. J. Rescue operation "turned a only rescuer "copyright© Murcia, 2006, RPI No. 08/2006/309

19. Pérez Vigueras, J. Perea Lifante, FJ. Campillo Pérez, J. I want to be firefighter - agenda of oppositions. Murcia. Ed. IFUR 2015.